HOME REMEDIES

Digestive System

Volume 1

Vaibhav Chawadre

Home remedies & natural treatments is simple enough... in fact, you'll probably find everything you need in your kitchen.

In the present times, natural cure home remedies are gaining momentum. Many people are heading their way towards adopting home remedy treatment to get rid of several forms of diseases. There is a natural home remedy for almost every ailment. The best part about them is that, they have no side effects and are absolutely inexpensive. Thus, not only are they safe for health, but also turn out to be an economical option. This trend for resorting to home remedies is not new. In fact, they have their origin in the ancient times. To deal with day-to-day problems, like cough and cold, headache, vomiting, upset stomach etc.; there are plenty of effective cure home remedies. Home remedy treatment makes use of things bestowed on us by nature like fruits, vegetables and herbs.

Table of Contents

Acidity

Acidity is the cause of surplus secretion of acid by the gastric glands of the stomach. Our stomach secretes an acid, which is necessary for the digestive process. This acid, in turn, produces various digestive enzymes, like pepsin, which help in the breaking complex food particles into elements that can be easily digested by the body. When there secretion of acid is more than necessary, it results in the feeling of immense heartburn, along with a sensation of inflammation in the throat. This condition has been given the name of acidity. Its other symptoms include formation of ulcers and dyspepsia. Consumption of alcohol, highly spicy food and Non-Steroidal Anti-Inflammatory Drugs (NSAID's) also trigger acid formation and result in acidity. Nonetheless, it can be cured at home using various procedures.

Acidity can be described as a condition wherein there is an excess of acid secretion by the gastric glands of stomach. Heartburn and gas formation are the major symptoms of acidity. Our body produces acid to digest the food we eat. However, problem strikes, when it produces more acid than what is required. It is, then, that the gastric juices move from the stomach, into the lower esophagus, making it dysfunctional. There are a number of reasons that lead to the formation of acidity. In the following lines, we have listed the causes as well as the symptoms of acidity. Read on to know about some home remedies for curing acidity.

Causes of Acidity

➢ *Excessive smoking*

➢ *Drinking too much alcohol*

➢ *Gastro duodenal (peptic) ulcer*

➢ *Hyper secretion of hydrochloric acid*

➢ *Reflux of gastric acid*

➢ *Not having meals on time*

➢ *Eating fried and spicy food on a regular basis*

➢ *Problems in the functioning of digestive system*

➢ *Being on an empty stomach for a long time or skipping breakfast*

➢ *Eating foods rich in fats, like chocolates*

➢ *Pregnancy*

➢ *Aging*

➢ *Obesity*

➢ *Excessive exposure to sun and heat*

➢ *Inappropriate food habits*

➢ *Negative emotions*

➢ *Weakness of the valves*

Symptoms of Acidity

➢ Burning sensation or pain in the stomach, 1-4 hours after a meal

➢ Chest pain

➢ Prolonged heartburn

➢ Inflammation in chest

➢ Feeling hungry frequently

➢ Constant pain in the upper abdomen

➢ Belching

➢ Nausea

➢ Bitter taste in mouth

➢ Loss of appetite

➢ Respiratory problems

➢ Vomiting

➢ Coughing

➢ Gastro-oesophageal reflux

➢ Voice change and formation of ulcer in esophagus

➢ Pain during muscular contractions

➢ Pain in ears

Home Remedies for Acidity

- If you are suffering from acidity, try to suck on a piece of clove. It will bring immediate relief.

- For people who are prone to acidity, intake of milk or other dairy products will prove to be helpful.

- Regular consumption of fresh mint juice can also help you get rid of acidity.

- Add two teaspoons apple cider vinegar and two teaspoons honey to a glass of water. Drink this concoction after meals, as it reduces the chances of acidity.

- Boil cumin seeds in a glass of water. Let it cool down and supplement your meals with it.

- Banana, cucumber and watermelon have been found to be helpful in treating acidity naturally.

- If you are have acidity problem, avoid taking tea, coffee and other aerated drinks. Instead, go for herbal tea, containing spearmint (pudina) and liquorice (mulethi).

- The simplest of all remedies is to have a glass of warm water every day, early in the morning. Water is believed to neutralize acidity.

- Drink coconut water 3 to 4 times in a day. It will help bring relief from acidity.

- If you are looking for an immediate relief, have a bowl of yoghurt. It is one of the most effective home remedies for acidity.

- If you constantly suffer from acidity, suck on 10 grams jiggery every day, after meals. It will help you avoid acid formation.

- Have a glass of cabbage juice every day, in order to avoid acid formation and the resultant acidity.

- If you want instant relief from acidity, take a glass of water with a teaspoon of soda in it.

Anorexia

One of the common eating disorders prevalent in the society today, anorexia nervosa is a condition in which a person has intense fear of putting on weight. Some of the other prominent characteristics of the disease include extreme low body weight and body image distortion. A psychiatric illness, anorexia makes a person limit his/her food intake and long to become severely thin. Such people voluntarily starve themselves, which, at times, also leads to death. Anorexia is mostly seen in adolescent females, but males cannot be ruled out of the illness completely. In the following lines, we have provided some of the major causes and symptoms of anorexia nervosa.

Anorexia nervosa, more popularly known as Anorexia, is an eating disorder that is usually associated with women. Although, in today's world, men are no exception to this disorder, it is more profoundly seen in women or girls. The disorder usually starts in the teenage years. An eating disorder, it is characterized by low body weight and body image distortion. The person suffering from it has an obsessive fear of gaining weight. Anorexia nervosa is a psychological problem that may be caused due to cultural pressure, family environment, genetic factor, etc. However, if detected on time, it can be treated using some home remedies. Know more about the natural ways of treating anorexia, all of which mainly involve stimulating the appetite.

Causes of Anorexia

- Low self-esteem
- Biochemical factors
- Psychiatric disorders
- Social pressures
- Genetic predisposition
- Cultural pressures
- Psychological issues
- Family environment
- Life transitions
- Perpetuating factors
- Stress and strain
- Emotional disturbances
- Chemical imbalance in the brain

Symptoms Of Anorexia

➢ Refusal to eat

➢ Insomnia

➢ Distortion of body image

➢ Excessive importance placed on body composition or shape

➢ Denial of seriousness of low weight

➢ Intense fear of gaining weight or becoming fat, even if the person is considered underweight

➢ Confused thinking

➢ Ritualistic eating (including cutting food into a planned number of bites)

➢ Spitting out food before swallowing

➢ Paying great attention to nutrition labels

➢ Major increase in exercise output, even when exhausted

➢ Hatred of foods that used to be favourites

➢ Increased or unnecessary use of laxatives

➢ Vomiting after eating (for the binge eating/purging subtype of anorexia)

➢ Weight loss

➢ Amenorrhea or interruption of the menstrual cycle

➢ Bone loss (osteoporosis or osteopenia)

➢ Extra sensitivity to cold

➢ Bloated stomach after eating (since the stomach loses its ability to deal with a normal quantity of food at one sitting)

➢ Yellowed and dry skin

➢ Thinning hair

➢ Irregular heart rhythms

Home Remedy for Anorexia

➢ If you are a victim of anorexia, the best way to cure it would be to take the ginger and rock salt treatment. Take a small piece of ginger and peel of its outer layer. Grin it and add a few drops of lemon, pinch of asafoetida and one black pepper, to form a paste. Have this paste in the morning, on an empty stomach, for about 15 days. It would work as an appetizer.

➢ A simple remedy for treating anorexia comprises of consuming about 2 to 3 oranges per day. Oranges help increase the appetite in a person.

➢ Apples also work as efficient appetizers. Apart from providing iron to the body, they also stimulate the appetite.

➢ Yet another simple method would be to boil water and add 2 to 3 cloves in it. Also add ½ tsp lime juice. Cool it down a bit and drink. Continuous drinking of this decoction, at least for a week, is likely to boost the craving to eat.

➢ Garlic proves effective in curing Anorexia nervosa. You can consume it in salads, soups or other preparations. Garlic stimulates digestive powers and is great for increasing appetite as well.

➢ Soups increase the appetite of a person. Vegetable soup, with pinch of rock salt and black pepper, would act as an efficient appetizer. For non-vegetarians, chicken soup would be beneficial.

➢ Eat salad 10 minutes before having your food. This may comprise of cabbage, tomatoes, cucumbers, beets and capsicums. Sprinkle a little rock salt and squeeze half of the lemon on it, along with a pinch of black pepper.

➢ Prepare dough with flour and sour grape juice, adding a pinch of rock salt. Make chapattis out of this dough. They will enhance the appetite of person, thereby helping cure anorexia.

➢ It is also believed that spicy food increase one's appetite. Have spicy food twice or thrice a week. It would help improve your appetite.

➢ Consume tomatoes, preferably raw. You can also use them, as an ingredient, in various preparations.

Intestinal Worms

Intestinal worms can be described as parasites that feed on the human body. They are mostly found in the gastro-intestinal tract of a person, primarily on the intestinal wall. Though everyone is susceptible to the disease, it is more often found in children. In fact, at a single time, they can be infected with more than one type of worms. Intestinal worms mostly strike during the rainy season. Though ingestion of undercooked meat, drinking infected water and skin absorption are the main reasons for their occurrence, there are a number of other factors also that lead to intestinal worms. In the following lines, we have listed the various causes and symptoms of intestinal worms.

The human body especially the stomach and the intestine is home to a number of parasites such as hookworms, roundworms, flatworms, etc. These parasites are helpful in the digestive process. However, at times, the parasites also create several problems. there are various causes for the problems caused - contaminated food, dirty fingers and food, faulty living, etc. some of the symptoms observed in people suffering from intestinal worms are diarihea foul breath, dark circles under the eyes, inflammation of the intestine and lungs, nausea, vomiting, anaemia and nutritional disorders, constipation and loss of weight. Intestinal worms can, nonetheless, be treated at home. In the following lines, we provide some home/natural remedies to cure/treat intestinal worms.

Causes of Intestinal Worms

- ➤ Eating contaminated food
- ➤ Dirty fingers
- ➤ Drinking contaminated water
- ➤ Walking bare foot
- ➤ Undercooked flesh foods
- ➤ Foods contaminated by dogs
- ➤ Faulty living style
- ➤ Transmitting agents, such as a mosquito
- ➤ Sexual contact
- ➤ Germs that enter through nose and skin
- ➤ Poor sanitation
- ➤ Using human excretion as fertilizer

Symptoms of Intestinal Worms

> ➢ *Diarrhea*
> ➢ *Foul breath*
> ➢ *Dark circles under the eyes*
> ➢ *Constant desire for food*
> ➢ *Restlessness at night, with bad dreams*
> ➢ *Anaemia*
> ➢ *Headaches*
> ➢ *Inflammation of the intestine and lungs*
> ➢ *Nausea*
> ➢ *Vomiting*
> ➢ *Loss of weight*
> ➢ *Fever*
> ➢ *Nervousness*
> ➢ *Irritability*
> ➢ *Constipation*
> ➢ *Cough*
> ➢ *Intense itching in the area around the rectum*
> ➢ *Weakness*
> ➢ *Immunodeficiency*
> ➢ *Swelling of facial features*
> ➢ *Chest pain*
> ➢ *Sweating*
> ➢ *Mental problems*
> ➢ *Lung congestion*

Home Remedy for Intestinal Worms

➤ *Ground some coconut and store it. Every morning, take a tablespoon of coconut at the breakfast. After three hours, take 30 to 60 ml of castor oil mixed with 250 to 375 ml of lukewarm milk. Repeat the process for a few days.*

➤ *Chewing three cloves of garlic every morning is likely to relieve a person suffering from intestinal worms.*

➤ *Grate a small cup of carrot. Have this early in the morning on an empty stomach. This is an effective way to treat intestinal worms.*

➤ *Extract fresh juice from an unripe papaya. Mix a tablespoon of this juice with three to four tablespoons of hot water. After two hours, have 30 to 60 ml of castor oil mixed in 250-375 ml of lukewarm milk. Repeat this for two days.*

➤ *Papaya seeds are also useful in treating intestinal worms. Powder the seeds and take 1 tsp of it with a cup of milk or water first thing in the morning.*

➤ *Papaya leaves are also beneficial in curing intestinal worms. Pour 250 ml of boiling water in a pan containing 15 gm of dry papaya leaves. Take this decoction with honey.*

➤ *Cut the bark of the pomegranate tree. Make a cold decoction of it and have it in the quantity of 90 to 180 ml three times a day. A purgative should be given after the last dose. For children, the quantity of this decoction is less - 30 to 60 ml.*

➤ *Take 1 tablespoon of a ripe pumpkin seeds. Before immersing in 250 ml of boiling water, peel and crush them.*

➤ *Powder the herb of wormwood and consume it in a dose of eight to sixteen gram doses daily. This is effective in treating in intestine worms.*

➤ *The oil of wormwood is also beneficial. Mix it with olive oil in the ratio of 1:8. Intake this in dose 50 to 100 ml.*

➤ *Alternatively, wormwood oil can be mixed with water for treating intestinal worms. In 120 ml of water, add 2 ml of wormwood oil. Give it as an enema for killing worms in the rectum.*

➢ *Mix equal proportions of the herb belleric myroblan and the seeds of the herb butea (palas). Have 1 tsp of this mixture 3 times a day.*

➢ *Consume 1 tsp of powdered seeds of butea every day to cure intestinal worms.*

➢ *Alternatively, the powdered seeds of butea can also be consumed in the form of a paste. Take 1 tsp each of powdered seeds of butea and honey and make a paste. Have this 3 times a day.*

➢ *Take the roots and bark of the vasaka tree. Prepare a decoction taking 30 gm of the root and bark in 500 ml of water. Boil this till the quantity reduces to 1/3rd. have 30 ml of this decoction two times a day for 2-3 days.*

➢ *A simple natural remedy would be to have a glass of boiled water with a tablespoon of rock salt. Have this empty stomach every morning.*

Indigestion

Indigestion, more popularly known as upset stomach, is a condition in which the stomach of a person finds it difficult to digest food. Medically known as dyspepsia, it is characterized by chronic or recurrent pain in the upper abdomen. It irritates the esophagus and leaves a bitter or sour taste in the mouth. Almost all the people have faced the problem of indigestion at some point of time in their life or the other. Though not a serious disorder, it needs to be treated properly, lest it turns into a chronic problem. To know more about the causes and symptoms of indigestion, read through the following lines.

Also known as dyspepsia, indigestion is a problem related to the stomach. It occurs when the digestive juices are not secreted properly as such resulting in uneasiness. Consuming a variety of food stuffs is one of the prime reasons for indigestion. Other causes are overeating, eating hurriedly without chewing properly, lack of exercise, improperly cooked food and also food allergies from beans, onions, seafood, etc. indigestion leads to pain in belly, nausea, bloating of stomach, uncontrolled burping, heartburn, flatulence and acid regurgitation. While indigestion occurs to men and women, its occurrence is more in females when compared to males. However, it is not a very serious problem and can be cured retreating to some home remedies. Learn to know how to cure indigestion naturally.

Causes of Indigestion

- ➢ Fast eating, without chewing properly
- ➢ Heavy meals
- ➢ Consuming excess alcohol
- ➢ Excessive smoking
- ➢ Pregnancy
- ➢ Peptic ulcer
- ➢ Stress and anxiety
- ➢ Anti-inflammatory drugs
- ➢ Changes in regular lifestyle
- ➢ Diseases that affect digestive organs
- ➢ Stomach cancer
- ➢ Gallstones
- ➢ Gastritis
- ➢ Skipping meals
- ➢ Wrong combination of food
- ➢ Inadequate secretion of stomach acids
- ➢ Certain diseases
- ➢ Improperly cooked food
- ➢ Lack of exercise
- ➢ Overeating

Symptoms of Indigestion

- ➤ _Pain in belly_
- ➤ _Nausea_
- ➤ _Bloating of stomach_
- ➤ _Uncontrolled burping_
- ➤ _Heartburn_
- ➤ _Flatulence_
- ➤ _Acid regurgitation_

Home Remedy for Indigestion

- A useful home remedy for treating indigestion would be to have half glass of pineapple juice after meals.

- In a glass of lukewarm water, add a spoonful of juice of lemon, one spoonful of ginger and two spoons of honey. Mix it well and drink. An effective remedy to cure indigestion.

- In a cup of hot water, mix a tablespoon of lemon juice. Have this mixture before meals. It would prevent any indigestion.

- It is recommended to apply some ice cubes over the stomach after meals. This would cure indigestion.

- Take equal parts of baking soda and water in a glass. Have this mixture. It would provide instant relief from indigestion.

- Add a tsp of cumin seeds in a glass of water. Drink this mixture.

- Consume a gram or two of the pulp of the belleric myrobalan fruit. This would ease and provide relief from indigestion.

- In a tsp of fresh coriander leaf juice, add a pinch of salt. Drink this two times a day.

- Alternatively, 1 or 2 tsp of coriander juice added to freshly prepared buttermilk is also effective in treating indigestion

- Eating half a tsp of aniseed is likely to be effective in treating indigestion.

- Take a tsp of ajwain and add a pinch of rock salt to it. Have this mixture for curing indigestion.

- Another effective remedy would be to chew a small piece of ginger sprinkled with salt for 5 to 10 minutes before meals.

- Intake a tablespoon of cinnamon water after one hour of having meals proves helpful in treating digestion problem.

- Consume 1 cup of ginger tea after food to solve the problem of indigestion.

- Having oranges and grapes would serve beneficially in curing indigestion.

- ➢ Add 2 to 3 drops of mint essence in a glass of water. Have this concoction every 3 to 4 hours to get relieved from indigestion.

- ➢ Take half a cup of Soya oil and add 2 to 3 drops of garlic oil. Massaging the stomach with this mixture is likely to bring relief from digestion problems.

- ➢ Prepare herbal tea using blackberry, raspberry, mint and chamomile. This would be useful in curing indigestion.

- ➢ Add a few drops of lemon or cider vinegar in a glass of water. Drink this mixture before meals.

- ➢ Consume a mixture of 1 tsp each of mint juice, lemon juice, and honey. This is effective in treating indigestion.

Stomach Ache

Rather than an ailment in itself, stomach pain, or abdominal pain, is more of a symptom, of some other disease. The person suffering from stomach ache faces tremendous pain in the abdominal part of his/her body. Stomach ache is one of the predominant symptoms found in majority of the disorders. It can range from being mild to moderate to severe. Stomach pain can affect anyone, irrespective of gender or age. There are different factors that contribute towards the pain. To know more about the causes of stomach pain, along with the symptoms, browse through the following lines.

One of the most common ailments, stomach ache can be experienced anywhere in the area that falls between the chests and groin. This pain can vary from being mild to moderate and severe. Men, women and children, all are susceptible to stomach pain. Some of the major causes of the ache are chronic constipation, indigestion, excessive gas, food poisoning, ulcers, appendicitis, and inflammation of the gallbladder, kidney stones, urinary tract infections and hernia. In the following lines, we have provided some home remedies for curing stomach pain.

Causes of Stomach Ache

- Jaundice
- Menstruation
- Excessive gas formation
- Indigestion
- Chronic constipation
- Ulcers
- Food poisoning
- Viral gastroenteritis (stomach flu)
- Appendicitis
- Inflammation of the gallbladder
- Food allergy
- Hernia
- Kidney stones
- Urinary tract infections
- Pancreatitis
- Upset stomach
- Stomach ulcer
- Irritable bowel syndrome
- Food poisoning
- Gas
- Abdominal disorders

Symptoms of Stomach Ache

- ➢ Loss of appetite
- ➢ Uncomfortable feeling in the stomach
- ➢ Vomiting
- ➢ Dysentery with blood
- ➢ Burning sensation in the stomach
- ➢ Urine and chest acidity

Home Remedy for Stomach Ache

➤ One of the most effective home remedies for stomach ache would be to mix 1 tsp each of mint juice and lime juice. To it, add a few drops of ginger juice and a pinch of black salt. Drink this mixture to alleviate pain.

➤ Grate a small piece of ginger and extract its juice. Apply this juice on the bottom of the belly and massage it gently. This will be effective in curing stomach ache.

➤ If the stomach ache is due to acidity, the best bet would be to drink plain soda water. It would provide instant relief from the pain.

➤ In 50 ml water, mix 2 tsp lemon juice and 1 gram rock salt powder. Have this mixture three times a day.

➤ Take dry ginger, black pepper, roasted cumin seeds, dry mint leaves, coriander, asafoetida, garlic and rock salt in equal quantities. Grind them well and make a fine powder. Have 1 tsp of this mixture, along with a glass of warm water, after meals.

➤ Taking three grams each of carom seeds and rock salt or common salt, along with a glass of warm water, helps in relieving a person from stomach ache.

➤ In half a cup of warm water, add a tsp each of ginger juice and castor oil. Have this mixture two times a day, to get relief from stomach ache.

➤ In a cup of water, add 20 grams aniseeds. Keep it overnight and strain the mixture the next morning. Drink it to get relief from pain.

➤ Mix one gram of rock salt and two grams of dried and crushed celery leaves. Eat it to get instant relief from stomach ache.

➤ Grind three grams of tender tamarind leaves, with enough water, to make a paste. Once it turns into a liquefied form, add a gram of rock salt. Drink this mixture to get relief from stomach ache.

➤ Combine 2 tsp lemon juice and 1 tsp ginger juice. Add ¼ tsp sugar to this mixture and have it two times in a day.

- ➢ Pomegranates are helpful in treating stomach ache. In a bowl of pomegranate seeds, sprinkle some salt and black pepper. Eat the seeds, while making sure to chew them properly.

- ➢ Grind bael (Aegle marmelos) and form a pulp. Mix it in a glass of freshly prepared buttermilk. Stir it well before drinking.

- ➢ Prepare a paste of fenugreek seeds. Now, add this paste to a bowl of curd. This is one of the most effective ways to treat stomach cramps and pain.

- ➢ In half a litter of water, add 2 grams each of black currants and fennel seeds and keep it overnight. The next morning, mash the contents in water and add a gram of sugar. Have this concoction daily, in the morning, to get relief from chronic stomach ache.

Gastritis

Gastritis is a condition, wherein, there is an inflammation of the lining of the stomach. Gastritis strikes suddenly in some people, while others develop it over a period of time. Medically termed as dyspepsia, this ailment causes pain in the upper abdomen. Generally, the same bacterium that causes stomach ulcer is responsible for gastritis as well. Though it is not a very serious problem, if left untreated, it might create long-term problem. There are several reasons for gastritis to occur. In the following lines, we have provided some of the causes and symptoms of gastritis.

A swelling or an inflammation caused in the mucus membrane lining of the stomach is called gastritis. Gastritis can either be a mild or acute. In some cases, it can also be chronic or severe. The most common symptoms for gastritis are loss of appetite, nausea, vomiting, headache and dizziness. It also causes pain and discomfort in the stomach. The other symptoms include coated tongue, foul breath, bad taste in the mouth, increased flow of saliva, scanty urination, a general feeling of uneasiness, and mental depression. The best way to cure or treat gastritis would be to turn to the natural remedies. In the following lines, we provide the home remedies for treating the problem of gastritis.

Causes of Gastritis

- ➢ *Viral and bacterial infections*
- ➢ *Peptic ulcer disease*
- ➢ *Pernicious Anaemia*
- ➢ *High intake of spicy foods*
- ➢ *Junk food*
- ➢ *Food cooked in adulterated oil*
- ➢ *Unhygienic conditions*
- ➢ *Excessive consumption of caffeine*
- ➢ *Excessive intake of alcohol*
- ➢ *Stress*
- ➢ *Depression*
- ➢ *Digestive disorders*
- ➢ *Irregular or excessive eating*
- ➢ *Wrong combination of foods*
- ➢ *Habitual use of large quantities of condiments and sauces*
- ➢ *Prolonged tensions*
- ➢ *Certain drugs*
- ➢ *Bile reflux disease*

Symptoms of Gastritis

- *Pain in stomach and head*
- *Weakness*
- *Vomiting*
- *Lethargy*
- *Unwillingness to eat*
- *Problem in urinating*
- *Depression*
- *Heaviness in abdomen*
- *Pyrosis*
- *Constipation*
- *Diarrhea*
- *Sour tongue*
- *Thick coat of sticky material over the tongue*
- *Bad smell from mouth*
- *Gnawing or burning ache or pain (indigestion) in upper abdomen*
- *Nausea*
- *Loss of appetite*
- *Belching or bloating*
- *A feeling of fullness in upper abdomen after eating*
- *Weight loss*
- *Ulcers*

Home Remedy For Gastritis

- One of the simplest and effective home remedy to cure gastritis would be to take a tsp of ajwain with a pinch of salt. Gulp this mixture with a glass of lukewarm water.

- Coconut water also proves to be effective in treating gastritis. Take coconut water twice a day.

- Another good remedy for curing gastritis is to make a combination of 200 ml of spinach juice and 300 ml of carrot juice. Drink this combination once a day.

- Apply heat through hot bags or hot water bottle in an empty stomach. This is effective in curing the problem of gastritis.

- Intake half cup of potato juice before meals. It is a natural way to treat gastritis.

- Take a cup of hot water and put a half a tsp of liquorice root tea. Boil the water for about 10 minutes after which strain it. Drink this concoction when warm. Repeat this at least thrice a day.

- Increase in the consumption of water and juices also helps to get relieved from gastritis.

- In 125 grams of curd, add 2 grams of Sprague and half gram of black salt. Have this mixture as it is effective in relieving gastritis problem.

- Combine Sprague powder and black salt in the ratio of 6:1. Intake 2 grams of this mixture, along with warm water. This is a good natural remedy to cure gastritis.

- Buttermilk and curd also works well to cure gastritis. Have buttermilk and curd along with asafoetida and cumin water.

- Take 2 teaspoons of peach leaves in a cup and add boiling water to it. After about 10 minutes, drink this concoction. Have this mixture thrice a day.

- Take a few figs and immerse it in warm water. After about 10 minutes, strain this water and drink it.

- Chew roasted fennel after meals. This provides relief from gastritis.

➤ *Intake a cup of rice gruel two times a day. This would impart relief from the problem of gastritis.*

➤ *Chewing fresh ginger before taking meals is also helpful in preventing and curing gastritis.*

Heartburn

Heartburn is a painful, burning sensation that occurs in the esophagus. Also known as pyrosis, the pain is experienced just below the breastbone and is mostly associated with the ejection of gastric acid from the mouth. Heartburn is usually caused in the chest region, but the pain may also subsidize to the other areas, such as neck, throat and jaw. Though termed as heartburn, the ailment is not associated with the heart by any chance. Stomach acidity is one of the primary reasons for heartburn. In the following lines, we have listed some more causes and symptoms of heartburn.

A burning sensation and pain in the stomach and chest region is termed as heartburn. Also known as pyrosis, it is generally a burning or painful sensation in the esophagus. This is caused due to the upward direction of gastric acid from the stomach to the chest. On its way up, the acid aggravates the tissues in the esophagus and the throat. Though termed heartburn, it is a digestive problem and is not concerned with the functioning of the heart. Eating fatty/oily foods, pregnancy, wearing extremely tight clothes, bending down, sleeping on a full stomach are some of the causes of heartburn. The symptoms of heartburn are bloating, gas, nausea, shortness of breath and/or an acidic or sour taste in the throat and mouth. However, heartburn can be treated at home using natural remedies. Learn to know how to cure heartburn naturally.

Causes of Heartburn

➢ *Alcohol consumption*

➢ *Excessive intake of caffeine*

➢ *Anti-inflammatory medications*

➢ *Carbonated beverages*

➢ *Acidic juices, such as grapefruit, orange or pineapple*

➢ *Acidic foods, like tomatoes, grapefruit and oranges*

➢ *Too much of chocolate*

➢ *Smoking*

➢ *Consumption of high-fat content foods*

➢ *Eating large meals*

➢ *A hiatal hernia*

➢ *Pregnancy*

➢ *Obesity*

➢ *Primary diseases of the esophagus*

Symptoms of Heartburn

➢ A burning sensation in the chest

➢ A burning feeling in the throat

➢ Sour or bitter taste in the mouth

➢ Belching

➢ Difficulty in swallowing

➢ Chronic coughing

➢ Loss of appetite

➢ Wheezing or other asthma-like symptoms

➢ Mild nausea

➢ Formation of excessive gas

➢ Fullness or heaviness in the upper abdomen

➢ Pain between shoulders or in neck, following food

Home Remedy for Heartburn

➢ On the first sign of heartburn, it is advisable to have water in larger quantities. This would work for those, whose symptoms are not too strong.

➢ An easy home remedy for heartburn would be to have half a tsp of baking soda in a glass of water. It is effective in treating heartburn.

➢ Combine 1 tablespoonful of apple cider vinegar, 1 teaspoonful of honey and 1 cup of warm water. Having this mixture would provide relief from heartburn.

➢ Consuming buttermilk during heartburn would bring in relief. It works very well for the ailment.

➢ Cinnamon is useful in treating heartburn. Make tea using cinnamon sticks. Have this tea once or twice a day. Another way to have it would be to prepare cinnamon sandwich.

➢ In a cup of water, add 1 ½ tsp of ginger root. Simmer this for about 10 minutes. Intake this drink as it would bring in relief for the pain.

➢ In a pan of 1 cup boiling water, put a tablespoon of the dried marshmallow root. Cover the pan with a lid and allow it to simmer for 15 minutes. Strain this liquid and have at least 3 - 4 cups per day.

➢ Drinking Aloe Vera juice acts beneficially in healing intestinal tract and thus relieving a person suffering from heartburn.

➢ Take 1 or 2 raw potato and wash them well. Do not peel, instead, cut them into pieces and churn them. Drink the juice immediately. The other option would be to mix it with some other juice for taste. However make sure that it is drunk instantly.

➢ Prepare tea using chamomile tea. Intake this tea after meals. This would relieve a person from oesophageal irritation.

➢ Take 1 tsp of yellow mustard with about ½ glass of water. This would stop heartburn instantly.

➢ *Take a cabbage and cut it into pieces. Immerse this in a pot of water and let it cook for about 7 minutes. Thereafter, add some mashed potatoes and a little olive oil. Have this mixture. It would heal the sensation of heartburn.*

Constipation

A problem of the digestive system, constipation affects people who have infrequent bowel movements, pass hard stools or strain during bowel movements. Constipation is wrongly anticipated as a disease. Rather, it is a symptom of many other diseases. People who suffer from constipation generally have painful bowel movement and often experience straining, bloating and sensation of a full bowel. Although it is not a serious ailment, constipation, if left untreated, can lead to serious problems. Read on to know more about the causes and symptoms of constipation.

Constipation is a problem of the digestive system. It gives rise to occasional bowel movement, incomplete evacuation of bowel, decrease in the volume or weight of the bowel. Not only is constipation a problem in itself, it is also the cause of many problems which occur due to it as toxins find their way into the bloodstream throughout the body. Some of the diseases caused due to it are appendicitis, rheumatism, arthritis, high blood pressure, cataract, and cancer. Some of the causes of constipation are low fibre diet, low intake of fluids, weak abdominal muscles and high intake of refined foods. When it comes to treating the ailment, the best way to do it is through the home remedies. Apart from solving the ailment, home remedies also add the required nutrients and have no side effect. Look out for some natural remedies to cure constipation.

Causes of Constipation

- ➤ Overeating/ having heavy meals
- ➤ Low fibre diet
- ➤ Low intake of fluids
- ➤ Lack of salads and fruits in diet
- ➤ Diseases like hyperacidity, diabetes, colitis, sluggish liver and tumours
- ➤ Weak abdominal muscles
- ➤ Holding back stools, when in pressure
- ➤ Irregular meals
- ➤ Incomplete chewing of food
- ➤ High intake of refined foods
- ➤ Faulty style of living
- ➤ Unhealthy eating habits, including intake of refined and fatty foods
- ➤ Insufficient intake of water
- ➤ Excessive consumption of tea and coffee
- ➤ Insufficient chewing of food
- ➤ Wrong combination of foods
- ➤ Lack of exercise
- ➤ Emotional stress

Symptoms of constipation

- Irregular discharge of stools
- Depression
- Bad breath
- Insomnia
- Pimples
- Heart burn
- Difficulty in eliminating feces
- Coated tongue
- Foul breath
- Headache
- Depression
- Insomnia
- Loss of appetite
- Dark circles
- Dizziness
- Acne
- Mouth ulcers
- Acidity

Home Remedy for Constipation

➢ *The most simple and effective home remedy for curing constipation is to have at least 6 to 8 glasses of water. This is beneficial for digesting and dissolving the nutrients.*

➢ *Consuming 2 tablespoons of molasses before going to sleep is a good remedy for treating constipation. You can also add it to milk, fruit juice, or prune juice if you want.*

➢ *Cabbage juice also is beneficial in treating constipation. Have half cup cabbage juice two times a day to counter constipation problem.*

➢ *Immerse 10 to 12 dry grapes without seeds in milk and heat the milk till it boils. Strain the milk. While you are drinking the milk, chew the grapes side by side. It is one of the useful remedy for treating constipation naturally.*

➢ *An effective method would be to immerse 5-10 grams Spiegel seeds in 200 grams of warm milk. Add sugar to it and drink this before going to sleep. Another way of using Spiegel seeds would be to soak 2 tsp of them in water for about 6 hours. Add equal amount of sugar to the mixture. Before going to bed at night, have this mixture.*

➢ *Keep water in a copper vessel overnight. Have this water first thing in the morning in an empty stomach. It is a useful remedy for constipation.*

➢ *In ½ glass water, mix ¼ tsp of Epsom salt. Drink this combination to cure constipation.*

➢ *A combination of orange juice and olive oil would also act beneficial to cure constipation. In ½ cup orange juice, add equal amount of olive oil. Drink this to get rid of constipation.*

➢ *Mix equal quantities of carrot juice and spinach juice in a glass. Intake this combination at bedtime. It would cure constipation problem.*

➢ *A before meal technique would be to have a tsp of linseed with water. It brings in the much needed lubrication required for constipation.*

➤ *Consuming hot water with sour lime juice and half a teaspoon of salt added to it would be beneficial in treating constipation.*

➤ *Orange juice when taken empty stomach in the morning would be favourable in treating constipation.*

➤ *Fennel seeds will help to cure the digestive problem. In a glass of lukewarm water add a few fennel seeds. Drink this mixture every night before going to bed. It would definitely heal constipation.*

➤ *In case of chronic or severe constipation, have figs dipped in water. Consume this in large quantities in the morning time.*

➤ *A guava a day in the early morning, keeps constipation away.*

Piles

Piles, also known as haemorrhoids, can be described as the swelling and inflammation of veins in the rectum and anus. There are two types of piles - internal and external. When struck externally, piles cause a lot of pain, but no bleeding. However, in case of internal piles, there is no pain, but a discharge of dark blood. Haemorrhoids are usually not dangerous or life threatening and in most of the cases, its symptoms will go away within a few days. To get information on the causes and symptoms of piles, go through the following lines.

Haemorrhoids, more popularly known as piles, can be described as a condition where the veins around the anus or lower rectum swell or get inflamed. It is due to this that a person faces difficulty in passing stool. Piles can be dry as well as bleeding. Even dry piles can result in bleeding, if they continue for a long time. There are two types of piles - internal piles, not seen but felt, and external piles, visible around the exterior of the anus region. Increased pressure from the internal or external veins can be one of the reasons of piles. Some other causes include low fibre diet, pregnancy, aging, hereditary factors, chronic constipation and anal intercourse. Piles can be treated using some home remedies as well. Read on to know some natural ways of curing haemorrhoids, or piles, at home.

Causes Of Piles

➢ *Chronic constipation*

➢ *Bowel disorders*

➢ *Prolonged periods of standing or sitting*

➢ *Obesity*

➢ *General weakness of the body tissues*

➢ *Mental tension*

➢ *Heredity factors*

➢ *Dysentery*

➢ *Hormonal changes during pregnancy*

➢ *Strenuous physical exercise*

➢ *Prostate problems in older men*

➢ *Straining, to empty the bowels*

➢ *Eating a low-fibre diet*

➢ *Chronic diarrhea*

➢ *Cancer or growths in pelvis or bowel, which puts pressure on abdomen*

Symptoms Of Piles

- Pain or irritation while passing stools
- Bleeding
- Slight bleeding, in case of internal trouble
- Feeling of soreness
- Irritation after passing a stool
- Itching
- Discomfort
- Pain in the rectal region
- Lump on the anus
- Pain and discomfort after you opening the bowels
- Slimy discharge of mucus
- Feeling that the bowels haven't emptied completely
- Soiled undergarments
- Swelling protruding from the anus
- Frequent urge for evacuation
- Loss of appetite
- Yellowish face, due to extensive bleeding
- Heaviness at the opening of anus

Home Remedy For Piles

➤ The best way to treat piles at home would be to have a mixture of yoghurt and black mustard. In a bowl of yoghurt, mix some powdered black mustard. While having it, make sure to chew the mustard very carefully. After this, drink a glass of buttermilk.

➤ In a bowl of water, soak peels of a pomegranate. Place the bowl on flame and let this water boil. Turn off the flame, strain the concoction and let it cool down. Drink this once in the morning and once in the evening.

➤ Prepare some buttermilk, using cow's milk. Add peppercorns, ginger and rock salt to this. Have this mixture two times a day.

➤ Put 10 gm black mustard in 150 ml goat's milk. In this, add 5 gm sugar. Drink this mixture in the morning, every day.

➤ In a bowl of yoghurt, put a few flowers of tamarind plant and some pomegranate juice. Once you have blended this well, add coriander and ginger pastes to it. Consume this after lunch. It will help pacify the pain.

➤ Grind some dry slices of yam into a powder. In 160 grams of this powder, add 80 grams white leadwort. Now, add 10 grams black pepper and 500 grams of jiggery. Mix well and make small tablets or capsules of this mixture. Have one piece each in the morning and evening.

➤ For bleeding piles, keep 1/4 litter goat's milk for curdling overnight. In the morning, add an equal amount of carrot juice and blend it. Drink this mixture. Alternatively, freshly prepared goat's milk yogurt, consumed with freshly chopped carrots, is also beneficial in treating piles.

➤ Radish is effective in curing piles. Extract the juice of white radish and mix it with honey. Apply this mixture on the affected region. This will prove helpful in treating piles.

➤ For instant relief, applying coconut oil on the affected region will be your best bet.

➤ Extract the seeds of ripe mangoes and dry them in the sun. Once dry, grind them into a fine powder. Store this powder in bottles.

Consuming 2 gm of this powder, with honey, twice a day will be effective in curing piles.

➢ *Mix ½ tsp each of ginger juice, lime juice and mint leaves juice, in 1 tbsp. honey. Have this mixture once a day. It will be helpful in treating piles.*

➢ *Take 1 tbsp. each of roasted black cumin seeds and cumin seeds (not roasted). Mix this well and add to a glass of cold water. Drink this concoction once every day.*

➢ *In a cup of milk, mash a ripe banana. Have this mixture 3 to 4 times in a day, to stop the pain experienced during piles.*

➢ *Soak 3 to 4 figs in a glass of water and keep them overnight. Have them early in the morning, on an empty stomach.*

➢ *Extract the juice of bitter gourd leaves. Mix 2 tsp of this juice in a glass of buttermilk and have it on an empty stomach, every morning.*

➢ *Extract about 150 ml of turnip juice. Consume this juice after combining it with any other vegetable juice, such as spinach, watercress or carrots.*

Urinary Tract Infection

Our urinary system comprises of kidneys, ureter, bladder and urethra. A bacterial infection that affects the urinary tract of a person is known as urinary tract infection (UTI). Though the infection can affect any part of the urinary system, it is usually the lower urinary tract i.e. the urethra and the bladder that is most affected by it. Women are more susceptible to UTI than men. Although it is painful and discomforting, urinary tract infection can be quickly and easily treated. Read on to know more about the causes of UTI, along with its symptoms.

An invasion of bacteria into the urinary tract causes UTI (Urinary Tract Infection). The bacteria enter from the opening of the urethra and proceed further into the urinary tract. Some of the causes of UTI include sexual intercourse, multiple sexual partners and holding urine for too long. Urinary tract infection can be very painful, if not treated in time. It can also spread to the kidney, causing serious health problems. Though the disease can affect members of both the sex, women are more susceptible to it. Some of the common symptoms of urinary tract infection are burning sensation while urinating, a constant urge to urinate, blood in the urine, fever, vomiting, nausea, backache and pain below the ribs. In the following lines, we have provided some of the best home remedies for treating UTI.

Causes Of Urinary Tract Infection

- ➢ Bacteria in the urethra
- ➢ Sexual intercourse
- ➢ Having multiple sexual partners
- ➢ Holding back the urge to urinate
- ➢ Prolonging urination
- ➢ Abnormal structure of the bladder
- ➢ Failure to empty the bladder completely
- ➢ Sexual positions
- ➢ Tumour in the urinary tract
- ➢ Stones in the urinary tract

Urinary Tract Infection

> ➤ *A burning sensation on passing urine*
>
> ➤ *Passing urine more frequently than usual*
>
> ➤ *Sensation of needing to pass urine, but being unable to do so*
>
> ➤ *Blood in the urine*
>
> ➤ *Feeling unwell*
>
> ➤ *Fever*
>
> ➤ *Chills*
>
> ➤ *Nausea*
>
> ➤ *Vomiting*
>
> ➤ *Tender or heavy belly*
>
> ➤ *Cloudy or foul-smelling urine*
>
> ➤ *Pain on one side of the back, under the ribs*

Home Remedy For Urinary Tract Infection

➤ Baking soda is effective in curing urinary tract infection. In an eight ounce glass of water, add ½ tsp of baking soda. Mix this well and drink it.

➤ Have plenty of water in a day, as this would help in diluting and flushing out the unwanted substances from the body.

➤ Drinking cranberry juice is another effective way to treat urinary tract infection. For people who cannot have pure cranberry juice, mixing it with some apple juice is an option.

➤ Mix equal proportions of sandalwood, bergamot, tea tree, frankincense and juniper oil. Rub this combination of oil in the abdominal area once a day, for three to four days.

➤ Mix equal parts of pipsissewa, buchu, echinacea and urva ursi tinctures. Have 20 drops of this mixture, every two hours, for the first two days and 1 tsp of this mixture, four times a day, later on.

➤ Another useful remedy for UTI would be to boil the leaves of blue brinjal plant in water. Cool the decoction, strain it and have an ounce of it two times in a day.

➤ Boil some coriander seeds in water. Cool the decoction, strain it and have an ounce of it two times in a day. It will increase the urine flow.

➤ The seeds of carrot are useful in treating urinary tract infection. They can either be taken as an infusion or as a decoction.

➤ In a bowl of water, put some petals of lotus and pink rose and bring it to boil. Strain the liquid after it cools. Have an ounce of this, three times a day.

➤ Chameli plant decoction is helpful in curing urinary tract infection. In a bowl of water, put Chameli plant and bring it to boil. Allow it to cool. Strain the liquid and drink it once daily

Peptic Ulcer

Peptic ulcers are sores that appear on the inner lining of the stomach, upper small intestine or esophagus. Ulcers are, most commonly, the result of either an infection or long-term use of certain medications. Also known as ulcus pepticum or PUD, they cause excessive abdominal pain. Though small ulcers do not cause any major problem, the large ones may lead to bleeding. There are a number of reasons, which can cause peptic ulcer in a person. In the following lines, we have listed the various causes and symptoms of peptic ulcers. Go through them and increase you knowledge about the ailment.

The erosion caused in the inner lining of the stomach and intestinal tract has been given the name of 'peptic ulcer'. While the ulcer in stomach is known as gastric ulcer, the one in intestinal tract, or duodenum, is called duodenal ulcer. When gastric ulcer and duodenal ulcer are clubbed together, they are known as peptic ulcer. The main causes of peptic ulcers are hyperacidity, excessive intake of alcohol, overeating, high intake of spicy foods, food poisoning, and high intake of coffee, smoking and presence of helicobacter pylori. The symptoms of peptic ulcer include sharp and severe pain, along with discomfort, in the upper part of the abdomen. When a peptic ulcer develops, the stomach swells due to excessive flatulence, mental tension, insomnia and gradual weakening of the body. Peptic ulcer, however, can be treated at home using some natural remedies. Given below are some home remedies to cure peptic ulcer.

Causes of Peptic Ulcer

➢ *Hyperacidity*

➢ *Overeating*

➢ *Taking heavy meals*

➢ *Highly spicy foods*

➢ *Excessive intake of coffee*

➢ *Too much consumption of alcohol*

➢ *Excessive smoking*

➢ *Food poisoning*

➢ *Infections*

➢ *Stress*

➢ *Certain drugs*

➢ *Food poisoning*

➢ *Gout*

➢ *Emotional disturbances*

➢ *Nervous tension*

➢ *Presence of helicobacter pylori*

➢ *Non-steroidal anti-inflammatory drugs or NSAID*

Symptoms of Peptic Ulcer

➢ Sever pain

➢ Discomfort in upper part

➢ Blood in the stool

➢ Vomiting of blood, which may appear red or black

➢ Dark blood in stools or stools that are black or tarry

➢ Nausea or vomiting

➢ Unexplained weight loss

➢ Change of appetite

➢ Belching

➢ Heartburn

➢ General discomfort in the abdomen

➢ Bloating or fullness after eating

➢ Feeling sick

Home Remedy For Peptic Ulcer

➤ The most effective home remedy for treating peptic ulcer is to eat bananas every day. It is an excellent way to neutralize the hyperacidity of the gastric juices. Banana milk shake is also beneficial in curing peptic ulcer.

➤ Having cold milk, without sugar, is effective in reducing the acid, thereby providing relief from burning sensation one encounters in peptic ulcer.

➤ Prepare a paste of 10 grams drumsticks leaves and water. Mix this paste in half a cup of yoghurt. Have this mixture every day, to cure peptic ulcer.

➤ In 250 ml of water, soak 15 grams leaves of wood apple and keep it overnight. Strain this concoction in the morning and have it.

➤ Applying a hot pack over the abdomen region is one of the effective ways of curing peptic ulcer.

➤ Cabbage and carrot, when mixed as juices, have been found to be beneficial in treating peptic ulcer. In half a litter of water, boil 250 grams cabbage until it is reduced to half. In a similar way, prepare carrot juice. Now, combine 125 ml of each juice. Once cool, drink it two times in a day.

➤ Tea made from fenugreek seeds is effective in curing peptic ulcer. When coated with water, fenugreek seeds become slightly mucilaginous, which helps in treating the ulcer.

➤ Combining carrot juice with spinach (or beet) and cucumber is effective in treating peptic ulcer. You can either mix 300ml carrot juice and 200 ml spinach juice or combine 300 ml carrot juice and 100 ml each of beet and cucumber juice, to make 500 ml of juice. Consume this daily.

➤ Blanch 5 almonds every day and extract their milk. Drink this milk every day, as it provides protein and also binds the acid in stomach.

➤ Drinking raw goat milk is effective in peptic ulcers treatment. For best results, drink this juice three times a day.

➢ *Lime is beneficial in curing peptic ulcer. The citric acid and mineral salts present in it help treat the ulcer. You can either have lime juice or use it in salads.*

Vomiting

Forceful expulsion of the contents of one's stomach, through the mouth and sometimes through the nose, is known as vomiting. The other names for vomiting are throwing up, emesis and informally, barfing. The sensations that a person feels prior to vomiting is known as nausea. Though one may experience a nauseating feeling many times, it is not necessary that he/she would vomit every time. Right from the problem of gastritis to brain tumour, there are various factors that leads to vomiting. Browse through the following lines, to know more about the causes and symptoms of vomiting.

An ejection of food and liquids from the stomach, through the contraction of the stomach muscle, is called vomiting. Also known as emesis, vomiting leads to the expulsion of solids as well as liquids, from the stomach. There are many reasons for vomiting like overeating, drinking excessive alcohol, pregnancy, migraine, infections, flu, upset stomach, etc. At times, vomiting is also one of the symptoms for a major disease as well. Its own symptoms include increased saliva, dizziness, light-headedness, difficulty in swallowing food or liquid, changes in skin temperature and increase in the rate of heartbeat. In the following lines, we have provided some of the home remedies of curing vomiting.

Causes of Vomiting

➤ Gastroenteritis problem

➤ Headache

➤ Inner ear disturbance

➤ Certain medical treatments

➤ High levels of toxins in the blood

➤ Hormonal changes

➤ Diabetes

➤ Peptic ulcers

➤ Gastroesophageal reflux disease (GERD)

➤ Gallstones

➤ Overeating

➤ Drinking excessive alcohol

➤ Pregnancy

➤ Migraine

➤ Infections

➤ Flu

➤ Upset stomach

➤ Stomach virus

➤ Food poisoning

➤ Intestinal obstructions

➤ Chronic digestive conditions

➤ Stomach cancer

➤ Intestinal obstructions

➤ Kidney failure

➤ Cholera

Symptoms of Vomiting

> ➤ *Involuntary expulsion of food from mouth and nose*
> ➤ *Increased saliva*
> ➤ *Dizziness*
> ➤ *Light-headedness*
> ➤ *Difficulty in swallowing food or liquid*
> ➤ *Changes in skin temperature*
> ➤ *Increase in heartbeat rate*
> ➤ *Increased sensitivity to certain smells*
> ➤ *Changes in the taste of some foods*

Home Remedy For Vomiting

➤ One of the effective ways to cure vomiting would be to have ginger tea. Make sure it has less amount of sugar.

➤ Chilled lime juice also proven effective in treating vomiting. In a glass of cold water, squeeze 1 lime. Add sugar and salt to taste. Put in some ice, to chill it. Drink this mixture after every two hours.

➤ If the vomiting is due to excess intake of alcohol, eat a slice or two of bread slowly, so that it soaks the liquid.

➤ Do not eat any solid food until after 12 hours of vomiting. Instead, have loads of vegetable juices, water and other non-acid drinks. Then only, start having solid foods, such as mashed potatoes, rice and oatmeal.

➤ On a non-stick pan, heat 2 cardamoms. Once heated, crush them to form a powder and add a tsp of honey to it. Have this several times a day.

➤ Prepare a mixture by combining 1 tsp each of mint juice and lime juice, with 1/2 tsp ginger juice and a tsp honey. Have it 2-3 times in a day.

➤ Boil a cup of water and add a tsp of cinnamon or one cinnamon stick to it. Steep it for some time and strain the water. Now, add a tbsp. of honey, for sweetening it. Have this decoction 2-3 times in a day.

➤ Holy Basil, catnip and peach bark tea are helpful for treating vomiting. You can have them in any form you like.

➤ A tsp of onion juice, taken after every two hours, proves beneficial in curing vomiting.

➤ Mix ¼ tsp powdered ginger, 1 cup apple juice and ¼ cup water together. Blend the mixture well, until the ginger gets dissolved, and add enough ice to make it slushy.

➤ Mix 1 tbsp. each of apple cider vinegar and honey in a glass of normal water and drink it before going to bed.

➤ Put some cloves, cardamoms or a cinnamon stick in your mouth. This is an effective way to treat vomiting.

➢ Cut a lemon into two halves. Sprinkle some rock salt on one of its piece. Lick this piece till all the juice runs out.

➢ Boil ½ cup of rice in 1 to 1½ cup of water. When the rice gets cooked, strain the water and drink it. It will help cease vomiting.

➢ In taking half a tsp of grounded cumin seeds, along with water, is helpful in stopping vomiting.

➢ Avoid too much of oily, spicy food, heavy and indigestible food, when you are suffering from vomiting.

Flatulence

Emission of a mixture of gases from the anus, which creates sound and is often accompanied by a foul odour, is called flatulence. Popularly known as farting, flatulence, apart from causing discomfort and pain because of bloating, also causes social embarrassment. The symbiotic bacteria and yeasts present in the gastrointestinal tract, causes the production of these gases, which is also called flatus. Excessive eating is also one of the prime reasons for such pressures to erupt. To know more about the causes and symptoms of flatulence, go through the lines that follow.

Flatulence is the emission of gases present in the intestine. The mixture of gases 'flatus' is released under pressure and creates a sound accompanied by a foul odour. Apart from causing discomfort and pain due to bloating, it also causes social embarrassment. The most common symptoms of flatulence or more popularly known as gas are a feeling of bloating and discomfort, excessive expulsion of wind, belching and pain in the abdomen. The problem of flatulence is very common and usually due to dietary reasons. Problems in digesting certain types of food cause flatulence. While for some it might be due to lactose intolerance, the others may suffer it because of grain based food. Yet, others might suffer due to foods which are heavy in carbohydrates. Flatulence, however, is not a serious problem and can be cured using natural treatments. Know more about the home remedies for curing flatulence.

Causes of Flatulence

➢ Presence of excessive amounts of bacteria in the intestines

➢ Consumption of large amounts of fibrous foods

➢ Consumption of products that contain malt extracts

➢ Digestive disorders that affect the GI tract, such as gastroenteritis

➢ Irritable bowel syndrome

➢ Constipation

➢ Food prepared under unhygienic conditions

➢ Contaminated water

➢ High-fat diet

➢ Metabolic breakdown of sulphur-containing proteins and amino acids in the intestines

➢ Fat mal-absorption

➢ Swallowed air

➢ Breakdown of undigested foods

➢ Lactase deficiency

➢ Dark beer and red wine

➢ Starchy food, such as potato, corn, etc.

➢ Certain Medication/Drugs

Symptoms of Flatulence

➤ *A feeling of bloating and discomfort*

➤ *Excessive expulsion of wind*

➤ *Belching*

➤ *Pain in the abdomen*

➤ *Foul odour*

Home Remedy For Flatulence

➢ *Do not forget the basics of eating as this is the most natural and effective way to treat flatulence. Eat slowly and chew the food thoroughly. Do not gulp the food. This is the best way to cure the problem of gas.*

➢ *In a cup of warm water, add 1/2 tsp of dry ginger powder with a pinch each of asafoetida and rock salt. Drink this mix to get relieved from gas.*

➢ *Take a cup of lukewarm water and add 2 tsp of brandy. Intake this before going to bed.*

➢ *Soak some ginger slices in lemon juice. Chew this after every meal. This would help cure gas.*

➢ *In a tsp of honey, add a drop of dill oil. Intake this after every meal to help treat flatulence.*

➢ *Grind 1 tsp of pepper, 1 tsp of dry ginger and 1 tsp of green cardamom seeds. Add ½ tsp of this mixture in water and drink it one hour after meal.*

➢ *Peppermint also proven effective in treating flatulence. Not only does it refreshes the breath, but also cures gas.*

➢ *Peppermint tea is also effective in treating flatulence. The other tea includes anise tea, spearmint tea, and caraway tea. Spearmint or peppermint candy would also do the trick.*

➢ *Avoid foods such as beans, cabbage, cauliflower, broccoli, yeast-containing foods such as breads and cheese. Carbonated drinks also produce gas.*

➢ *Do not drink water after 15 minutes or during meals. It weakens the digestive system.*

Health and Beauty Tips

Natural remedies are the best way to maintain your health and beauty, as opposed to harsh medications and cosmetics. The concept of beauty appeals to all of us and is something fundamentally human. Health and beauty go hand in hand, as good health is a guarantee for a healthy body. Here are some natural remedies that will help enhance your health and beauty.

Health Tips:

➢ *Adequate sleep is essential for good health. Get an average of 7-8 hours of sleep every day.*

➢ *If you can't exercise at a stretch, exercise in small intervals of one minute of high intensity running or stair climbing or jumping followed by 1 minute of slow relaxed walking or marching. Do it for 5-6 minutes 3 times a day.*

➢ *Jumping on a rebounder is a great exercise. It helps tone and tighten the body, enhances blood circulation, and reduces cellulite. It is also easier on the knee and ankle joints and hence a great option for people who suffer from joint pains but want to lose weight.*

➢ *Enrol in an exercise form like Pilates, traditional yoga, power yoga or aerobics. Alternatively enrol in a salsa class or kick boxing for added fitness.*

➢ *Kegel Exercises are great for strengthening pelvic muscles. They are recommended during pregnancy for ease of delivery.*

➢ *Deep breathing exercises work wonders for health. Practically all diseases are believed to be curable by practicing various deep breathing exercises on a regular basis.*

➢ *Extra Virgin Olive Oil is best consumed unheated. It is best to use it as a salad dressing instead of cooking with it. Drink 15 ml of Virgin coconut Oil twice a day for increasing BMR, battling thyroid and losing weight.*

➢ *Wheat Grass or Spirulina are great health tonics. Consume them once a day for total health rejuvenation*

➤ Substitute one meal with black beans and salad. Black beans provide roughage and proteins and keep you feeling fuller for a longer time.

➤ Avoid eating late at night. It's best to consume the last meal of the day by 7:00pm. Eating late or eating just before bed time does not give the body enough time to digest it. Also, since activity levels decrease with the passing day, less calories are needed and hence eating late at night risks the food being stored as fat instead of being utilized as energy.

➤ Opt for organic sesame oil or coconut oil as your cooking medium, as they are least prone to oxidation due to heat and retain almost all nutrients on heating even at a high temperature.

➤ 1-2 garlic pods chopped and swallowed with water first thing in the morning can keep heart ailments at bay, reduce cholesterol, increase BMR, and boost the immune system.

➤ Consume at least one cup of organic green tea a day.

➤ Apples are a great source of fibre. People suffering from constipation must include at least two apples a day. Sprinkle with psyllium husk for added roughage.

➤ String cheese, pickles, olives, and dried fruits make for healthy snacks instead of refined foods since they are low calorie foods, rich in proteins and good fats. They keep one feeling fuller for longer and hence help avoid binge eating.

➤ Calcium is one of the key ingredients for weight loss. Lack of calcium will deter any weight loss efforts. Include dairy products like milk, cheese, cottage cheese and yogurt for daily calcium requirement.

➤ Try using organic whole milk instead of the homogenized versions; the fresher the better.

➤ Ensure that that your intake of good fats like the Omega 3 fatty acids in adequate amounts. They help fight fat and keep the heart healthy. Rich sources of Omega 3 Fatty acids include wheat germ oil, walnuts, pumpkin seeds, purslane (dark, leafy green used throughout Mediterranean countries), hemp seed oil, flaxseeds and its oil.

➤ Organic foods are wholesome and nutritious as opposed to pesticide laden and genetically altered foods. Hence it is always advisable to opt for the organic varieties of foods.

➤ Refined foods contain high sodium levels and empty calories. Avoid them.

➤ Ensure that you get adequate proteins if you are a vegetarian. Pulses are an excellent vegetarian source.

➤ Skim milk is made by removing milk fat. The remaining milk is full of milk sugar or lactose and devoid of many nutrients. Lactose is a simple sugar and is responsible for massive weight gain. Instead of drinking skimmed milk, try diluting full fat or whole milk with water. Alternatively prefer 2% milk.

➤ Almost any dental ailment is known to be cured with gargling with organic sesame oil for 5 minutes for a few days.

➤ Stay clear of diet sodas and sugar free foods. They contain artificial sweeteners, which contain Aspartame. This causes insulin spikes, lowers blood sugar, and makes you hungrier.

➤ Aromatherapy and steam inhalation are great remedies that will rejuvenate and cleanse your respiratory system irrespective of your health status.

Beauty Tips:

➤ Splash water over your face at regular intervals for keeping the pores unclogged and the skin hydrated.

➤ Keep your skin well hydrated in both summer and winter. If you're allergic to any moisturizer, apply a mashed banana mixed with cream and honey. Rinse after 15 minutes.

➤ Castor oil is a great moisturizer. Apply some to the face and dry elbows, knees and heels and keep it overnight to soften them. Rinse with warm water in the morning.

- Add a teaspoon of olive oil to a warm bath during winter to prevent the skin from drying. Olive oil mixed with egg and lemon juice is a time tested face mask for younger and firmer skin.

- Salt, sugar, oatmeal, crushed almond, and gram flour, make for excellent scrubs. Mix with some cleansing cream or simply with milk or yogurt. Scrub the face in a gentle circular motion for removing dead skin cells.

- To combat greasy skin, make a paste of lettuce leaf, a small rose and lime juice. Apply over the face and keep it on for 15 minutes, before rinsing off.

- Cucumber is a good cooler and a cleanser. Cucumber juice is also a great astringent. Just dab it on before you leave the house to venture into the sunny outside.

- Olive Oil mixed with equal quantities of vinegar is an excellent remedy to remove a sun tan.

- A pinch of camphor powder mixed in coconut oil massaged over blemishes helps lighten them and in many cases completely obliterates them.

- Rubbing a raw potato slice over the eyes can help reduce dark circles.

- Tomato is known to obliterate blackheads. Rub a tomato slice over the corner of the nose and other areas prone to blackheads.

- Virgin Coconut Oil is one of the most effective oils in treating skin ailments and allergies. Psoriasis, eczema, and pigmentation, all find a remedy in Virgin Coconut Oil. It is an excellent moisturizer and a night repair treatment.

- Evening Primrose oil in capsule form is great for overall skin health.

- Ageing women often opt for electrolytic peel treatments. Instead opt for homemade peels. Try this peel mask: mix dried yeast, orange juice, raw milk and rose water in sufficient quantities. Apply on the face till it dries and rinse off with warm water. This is one of the most effective home peel treatments if done consistently twice a week.

- *Vitamin E is the secret to great skin. Include wheat germ in your daily diet for a daily dose of Vitamin E.*

- *Vitamin C enhances overall skin health. Consume Indian gooseberry to obtain your daily dose of Vitamin C.*

- *Daily intake of carrot, beetroot and celery juice can keep the skin looking radiant and young.*

- *Massage your lips using a soft toothbrush and any toothpaste. This is excellent for the removal of dead cells and improvement of lip tone.*

- *Half a lemon dipped in salt and rubbed over teeth is proven to polish dull teeth and whiten them.*

- *Mix iodine with olive oil and rub over finger nails to strengthen them and prevent flaking.*

- *Dull and damaged hair can be conditioned with the application of almond oil, left in overnight.*

- *Rinsing your hair with beer or vinegar helps soften rough hair.*

- *Henna and Indian goose berry are great for your hair. Powdered and mixed with water or yogurt, they nourish the hair and give it a natural colour.*

- *Always opt for herbal skin and hair care products since they have fewer side effects and the results last longer.*

- *Lastly a good night's sleep ensures that you wake up to a radiant and nourished skin in the morning.*

- *Lastly, your consumption of water is of the utmost importance so make sure you get the required amount. This amount may vary depending on your physical proportions, your region, and the climatic and weather conditions, but is generally around eight glasses.*

Note

This is a simple home based treatment book that assists to fight diseases with easy natural home based cures.

The content in the book is provided for the sole intention of educating people on topics regarding health and disease management. All information featured in the book, including information pertaining to health conditions and remedies, is for informative reasons only. No information in the book should be blindly followed. This book is not intended to be used for instructional medical diagnosis, first aid, treatment and emergency care. The information provided does not replace medical advice or personal counselling, at all times consult your family doctor prior to making a health decision.

This book offers information for symptoms and causes of medical conditions. Please do not rely only on any given information pertaining to symptoms and causes present in the book.

It does not necessarily imply that all symptoms may be present for a particular condition. The listed symptoms and causes are not essentially the most typical for a condition. Symptoms and causes may differ, or be missing, depending on the seriousness of the condition. Symptoms and causes may change after a while with the advancement of the conditions. Symptoms may change at various phases of the conditions.

Not all causes and symptoms would be applicable to all patients. A particular class of patients, including pregnant women, babies, children, aged, or those with other severe complications may go through different symptoms. Some symptoms could be hidden and difficult to identify or could be detected only by a medical professional.

This book bears information written or rendered by third parties. Any notions, advice, testimonials, or other information conveyed or created by third parties, are that of the third party, and does not assert or suggest those of Author. Hence, not responsible for accuracy, reliability or adverse reaction to any opinion, advice or content in the book.

ISBN-13: 978-1533023896
ISBN-10: 1533023891